SELF THERAPY FOR BEGINNERS

The cutting edge and easy guideline to create wholeness and heal your inner self by using effective psychotherapy remedies; Self-healing techniques for newbies that show results in less than 7 days

Part-2

BY

Tom Bhowey

Table of Contents

Intro to meditation

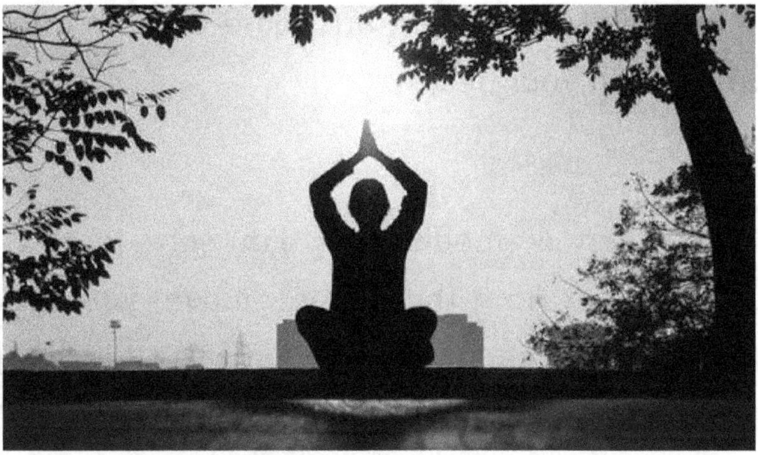

For hundreds of years, meditation has always been around. It has been deemed as a spirituality, so it can be challenging to become something of established scientific advantages.

But the reality is, meditation isn't just about connecting with and healing your soul! Meditation stimulates the mind as well as body with actual, physical consequences.

While a great deal of research already remains being done on meditation, there are some positive impacts it can have on your health.

So what then is meditation? I'm sure if you are reading this, or from the picture above, you already have a general idea in your head of what it is, but just to shed more light, Meditation is an activity which will train your brain to monitor and control itself.

It's the capacity to continually focus on one sort of stuff without cut in the process. When done consistently and diligently, it is a constant connection to your true inner selves.

Most individuals break away from the concept of meditation as we wonder, "How do we operate outside our ideas?" "How can we get thru our day without thinking?”

One aspect many people don't understand is as our bodies need regular exercise to keep our heads solid, fit and healthy.

Many times, whereas they underestimate this point, people ignore their minds. You're totally right if you find meditation as challenging. It's very frustrating to get your mind to shut down for five secs and don't talk of anything else.

That would be another cause why individuals don't attempt it. The very first moment I locked eyes to meditate, it did feel like any other single idea that I had have had all through my stay on the planet at that exact time chose to come into my mind.

They continued to come again, no matter which way I attempted to push it out, forget my emotions, or attempt to be in a state of banality.

During a break, the following time I sat to meditate, and so this moment my emotions dropped by a fifth. Throughout that retreat, the following which was the 3rd time I sat to meditate, they fell by half.

Steadily, it was as if I had begun to really see the Good-Definition universe. Not only did I perceive my external factors so plainly, but I ended up experiencing my innermost self with most of the objectivity that honesty I never had before.

Benefits of meditation

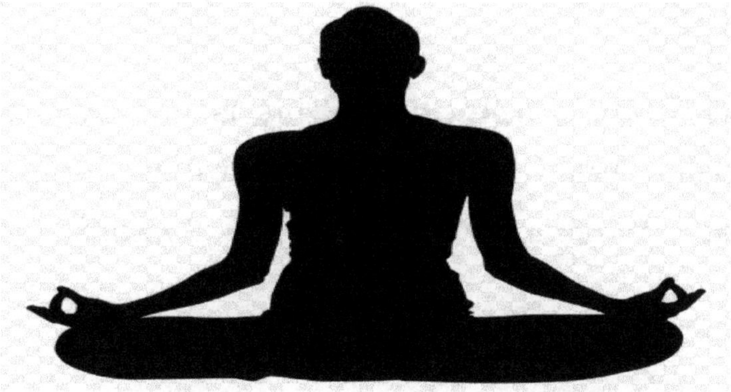

Relieve stress: stress can occur anywhere, even in a non-stressful situation, usually leading to panic attacks or wrong decision making.

When you feel stressed, you have a physiological reaction, which can negatively impact your health over the long term. Stress can cause headaches, aches and pains, anxiety, depression and a number of other physical symptoms.

Granting yourself a cut from stress's physical consequences can help relieve its symptoms aggravated by stress.

Boosts the body’s immunity: This is one of the most surprising health benefits of meditation. Stress And Anxiety Weaken Your Immune System By Causing Havoc.

Similarly to noticing thoughts and feelings of yourself, meditation gives you the possibility to look at memories you've got with others from a one of a kind attitude as well.

Improves self-assurance: on the memories you've got just yourself, your self-belief is hooked up.

And just as meditation helps you gain know-how of yourself, it also builds you via meditation. When a poor mind or emotions about yourself emerge, your goal to observe them in the meantime.

This lets in you to better control bad internal dialog outside of meditation over the years.

Exercise: the exercising of the frame, now not simply the exercising of the thoughts. You're given the capability to attend to yourself externally whilst you are taking care of yourself internally.

Improves creativity: creativity is a function of the brain's efficiency, the "geniuses" that we know of, who are masters of creativity in their fields, are people who have been able to utilize more percentage of their brains than the normal human being.

Even a small fraction matters. A number of significant & extenuating factors are behind the productive obstacles. Whichever the reason, the results are usually that you will get trapped in some thinking patterns, then you can't move beyond them.

As you're looking to go past one of these barriers it's like pressing the restart button to take time to relax. You always get out of those habits as you move away, allowing you to push past them.

Relieves pain: meditation is highly recommended by experts to those suffering from chronic pain, be it physical or emotional. Improves the overall performance of mind use: it's far no wonder that maximum mind output instruments are used as a shape of meditation.

Gives you compassion, tolerance, acceptance and willpower: being able to see everyone like their true selves because of reconnecting with yourself.

Meditation has a massive impact on your bodily health, but by helping improve your mind, it can additionally give you an intellectual enhancement.

Improves attention: it calls for attention to finish with gracefully any challenge at hand. Concentration is a key element for success, whether it is a scholarly feat or an expertise feat.

Meditation is absolutely a rest exercise! Whilst you discover ways to deal with your breath, notice whilst you get lost in your mind, and return your attention in your breath, and you could transfer that skill into any range of settings you choose.

Staying in the present moment: it's easier to live in the past, it's more fun to live in the future, but it's better to stay in the moment. And that's what meditation does for you.

Meditation helps to reduce high blood pressure: the majority of people who start practicing meditation regularly can actually lower their blood pressure so much, that they are able to stop taking blood pressure medication altogether.

This is because meditation helps promote relaxation and helps improve circulation. When this happens, the blood vessels open up and improve blood flow, therefore decreasing blood pressure. It is a natural as well as effective way to help alleviate a very serious condition.

Helps with addiction: Human beings who've extreme addictions, substance abuse issues, and who abuse alcohol can see brilliant results on their road to healing with regular meditation.

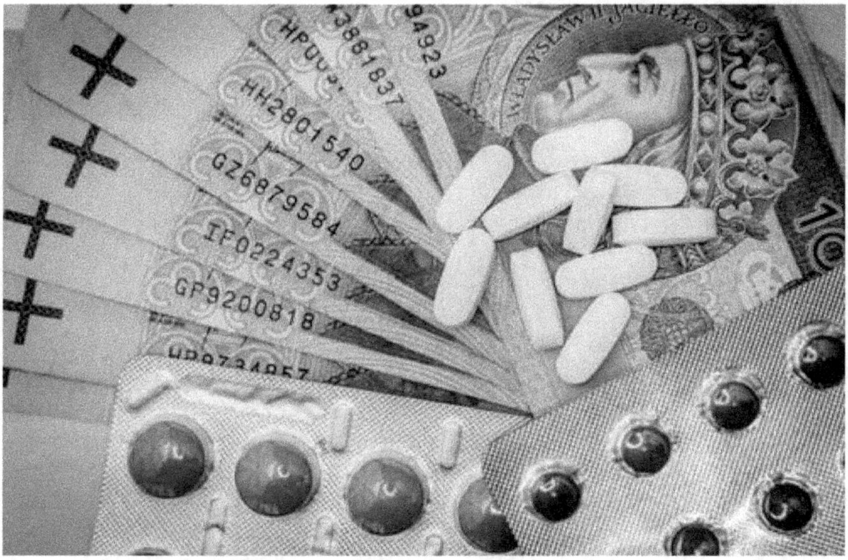

The pressure is one of the major factors that sound people are struggling with dependency to present good to their souls. Normal meditation combats stress, and the chain response can assist to get higher manipulation over addiction issues.

Attain wholeness of self (mind and body): The energy of spending even a few minutes an afternoon connecting with your body and your mind isn't always to be underestimated.

Doing so produces this innate experience of well-being that might be described as oneness, balance, or self-connection.

In a global environment where most of our time is spent specializing in outdoor events, it is possible to exchange our reviews in life for even a few minutes to reconnect with our inner feelings and sensations.

You might feel that you're too busy for something like meditation. But studies suggest that people with jam-packed schedules stand to benefit most from meditation!

The great thing about this is that is you can as well meditate for 5-10 minutes a day, which will also be beneficial to your psychology life. And still receive many of the amazing benefits that meditation offers so why not draft a routine and join the league of meditators.

The parts of meditation

There are three major aspects of meditation: approach, practice and integration

Approach

The approach is about how you view both the contents of your mind and the technique.

Get this right and your meditation will be great but make a mistake and you fall into an endless struggle. A mistake that first-timers make is thinking that they will get excellent results after meditating a few times.

The thing is that, like any other skill, you need a lot of practice to get the hang of it.

Firstly, you have to realize that your mind is not going to be in one place like the Zen masters in movies, and that is not the point, anyway.

The factor is to expand a new relationship together with your mind and emotions that permits effective feelings to unfold truly.

Skepticism is another thing that sets in easily, “of course it won't work for me” or “I’m not the meditation type”. When you meditate in the right way, it works for everyone. If you're cynical, fine.

But do attempt it anyway. Wouldn't it be satisfactory to be wrong about this? Other than impractical expectancies first-timers have, the largest impediment for the majority is making an attempt seem too hard for themselves.

That is one location to your existence wherein you sincerely shouldn’t conflict. In reality, applying masses of attempt is counterproductive. You're unfastened just to see what happens, isn't always that a comfort?

Practice

This is the second phase, this is where you actually do the meditation. There are a few steps laid down for you to try out.

Step one. Before you start

Before you start, you need to ensure that some things are in place. When are you going to have it done every day?

Where are you able to sit down undisturbed? How can you even don't forget to do it? The first step is committing to an ordinary, day by day exercise.

Taking five to ten minutes out of each day shouldn’t be difficult, but it’s easy to get caught up in everything that’s going on that we end up saying “I’ll do it tomorrow”.

Try and make it an everyday part of your time table. Create a space to take a seat at the identical time each day.

Mornings appear to paintings first-rate for the majority, other evenings, but you should pick a time frame that suits you.

It doesn't matter where you do it, just as long as it is unlikely that you will be interrupted. You also do not necessarily have to be in a yoga outfit or dressed up like a Chinese monk, just make sure that your outfit is free and will not disturb you during the process.

Step two. Settle down

For this second step, you need to find a quiet space where you can relax. Sit comfortably in a chair such that your hands are resting in your thigh or on your knees.

Keep your back straight, not leaning your back on the seat might come in handy for

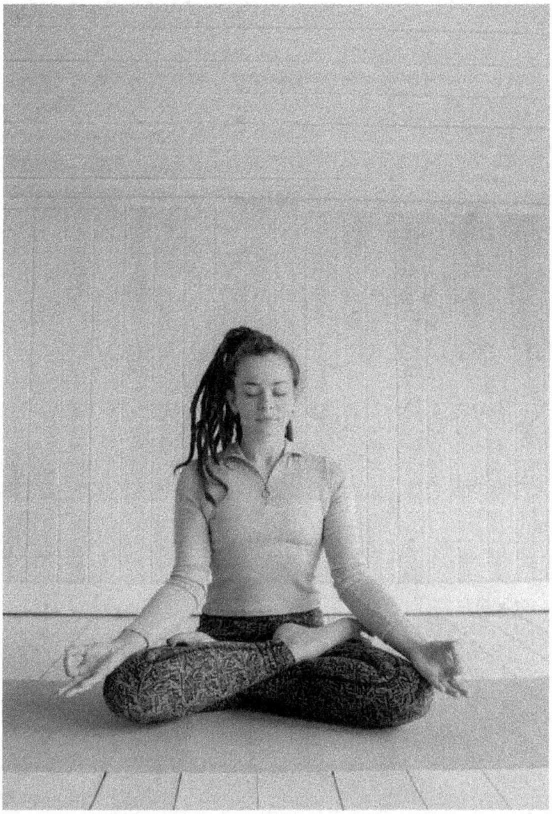

this stance. With your chin bent in a little bit, your neck must be relaxed too.

Whether you're using a timer or following meditation music, commit to practicing for the full time you've set aside, whether you find the session easy or difficult.

Step three. The breaths

Try not to focus your gaze on anything, like you are looking but not seeing. Some people just go for closing their eyes but if you want them open, fine.

Take seven deep, audible breaths, breathing in through the nose and exhaling from your mouth. On the final exhalation, let your eye lids to shut gradually.

Step four. Observe

Take some minutes to allow yourself to settle in then Have a look at your posture, and be aware of the sensations where your frame touches the chair, and your toes meet the ground.

Feel the weight of your fingers and palms resting on your legs, recognize your senses by noticing anything you can smell, hear or taste and sensations of heat, cold or wind.

Step five. Body scan

Just like a medical practitioner or a technician, you run diagnostics on your body by slowly turning your mind inwards.

You then do a mindful body scan from crown to sole, observing any tension or distress. Don't attempt to alternate what you find, actually take note of it. Test once more, although this time notice which components of the frame experience cozy feelings.

Take about 20 seconds for each test. Now deal with your mind. Word any thoughts that arise without attempting to regulate them.

Gently note your underlying mood, just turning into privy to what's there without judgment. Also, if you do not observe anything, it's okay.

Step six. The purpose

The next step is to pause for a while, about thirty seconds and identify the purpose of your meditation for that day. Recognize any expectation or desire you came with, and leave it to go.

Spread the affection: take a moment to consider the broader effects of being aware nowadays.

Feeling calmer allows you to experience better and the positivity is reflected on people you meet and interact with during the day, ranging from work colleagues to partners to your bus driver or office guard. Become aware of this ripple effect.

Also, before you continue in the session, remind yourself that there's no "thing" for you to do here, your only job is to sit for the full session, you are not fixing anything or looking for what needs fixing, all you have to do is sit back and relax and let everything unfold naturally.

Step seven. Keep tabs on your breathing

Pay close attention to the breathing process. Don't attempt to adjust it, only experience the rise and fall sensation in your system that it produces.

Notice where these sensations occur, it could be your belly, your elbows or wrists, fingers, ear, etc. for some moments, focus on the quality of each breath, noting whether it's deep or shallow, long or short, fast or slow.

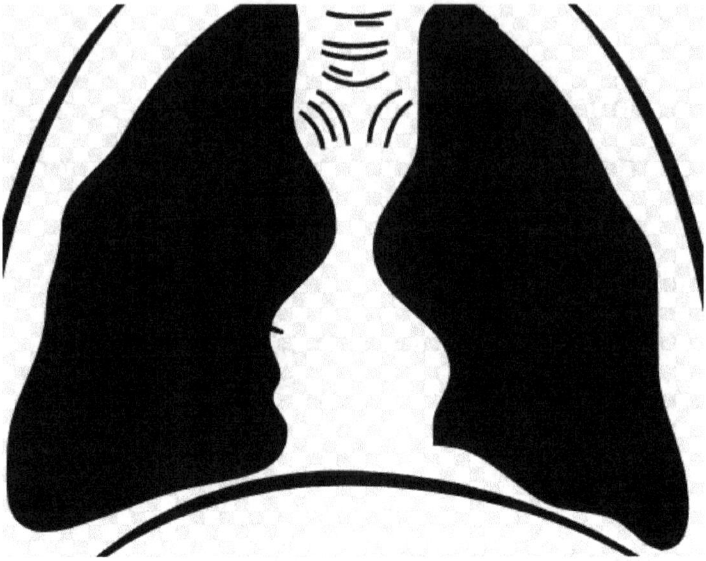

Count the breaths silently in this format; one as you inhale, two as you exhale, three on the next inhalation, and so on, up to ten. Then start again at one with the next inhalation.

If one to ten is too short for you, you can make it twenty.

This is the real concentration trainer, once you start this process, different thoughts start popping up, in an attempt to distract you.

When you realize that you have strayed, ward off those thoughts and go back to your counting. Unless you can know the exact number that you were adding up to, proceed again, or just resume from 1 again. Proceed till the countdown rings out.

Step eight. Allow your mind to be free

After the counting process, you should spend twenty to thirty seconds just sitting. You might find yourself overwhelmed with thoughts and plans, or feel calm and focused, it is usually common at this stage.

Whatever happens, it is completely fine. Enjoy the rare occurrence of letting your mind be.

Step nine. Preparing for the finish

Let your awareness find its way back to your physical feelings once more, feel The seat under you, whereby your feet comes into contact with just the board, hands and fingers placed in your lap.

Take note that anything you listen to, sense, taste or experience something. When you're comfortable open up your eyes gradually.

Step ten. On to the next

Now that you are done meditating and are about to leave the seat, do not just stand up and leave, focus on your next activity.

It could be to take your bath, eat your meal, etc. Try to carry this awareness with you to the next activity.

Referencing: Take small opportunities during the day to tell you how it is like to get that insight and focusing attention. Perhaps when you seat at your chair at work, during the drinking of your early coffee, even when you're in a taxi.

You shouldn't have to do each of the exercises, just take a couple of deep breaths, notice how you feel, and observe any areas of tension.

How to overcome potential obstacles during meditation

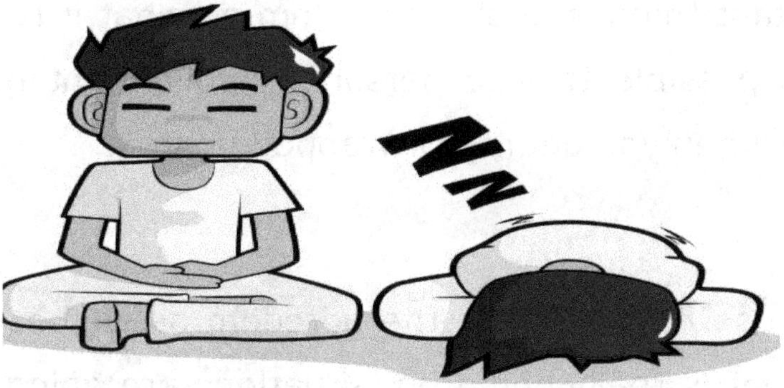

Everyone who learns to meditate encounters one distraction or the other during the course of meditation. Here are some of the most common challenges faced by meditators and a few tips on how to deal with them.

Boredom

A lot of people get bored at one point in time or the other during meditation, which is not surprising due to our busy, adrenaline-filled lives, characterized by raving and the internet.

The important thing is seeing boredom as what it is. It really is possible to lose personal involvement in meditation when you get really wrapped up in it.

But if you use it to examine the boredom as well as find out what is really going on, situations are going to keep getting exciting again.

You should not expect a lot from it like in the action movies where the protagonist does a dying minute meditation and gets enlightenment and strength to defeat the antagonist.

If you had your hopes up with respect to that, you will get bored. What you can do is to have this "surprise me" mindset before you start and you will find every result amazing.

Feeling sleepy

Some days are just fatigue days, no matter how you try to shake it off, you still feel tired. The key here is the basic anti-sleep techniques available out there like setting your alarm, ensuring you sit upright, you could also choose another time of the day if you realize that you usually get tired during the period you fixed for meditation.

Feeling scared

Sometimes the mind can be a dark and frightening place. Often sitting with hard thoughts and feelings will feel too much to deal with.

But as long as all this material stays unrecognized, in the background it just sits there. The first step of letting go of it and moving on is allowing it to come to the surface.

Feeling uncertain

"Is this strategy functioning? Do I get it straight? Perhaps I should only ..." Occasionally, skepticism eventually spreads.

But what occurs often is we fall into the uncertainty. We overlook that they're just words, no matter how much the emotions are.

The point is to realize when you've been distracted – no matter what the content of the thoughts – and to gently return your attention to the object of meditation.

Feeling agitated

You'll be relieved to know that almost everyone at first feels restless. This is generally because there's going to be a little too much energy trying to be still.

If you have to change your posture or have a scratch, feel free, just try not to move too much because it is difficult for the mind to settle down.

Feeling gloomy

Meditation's intention is to relax into a deep, fundamental sense of relief. But if you don't leap with joy out of your head, you don't do something wrong.

Sadness is a natural human emotion, and shedding a tear in contemplation is not unusual.

Honestly, there's almost something fun about it, maybe a feeling of letting something go.

Feeling lonesome

I have "things to do". This relentless diversion also keeps us from seeing how we really feel. If you sit to meditate, it can come to the surface, even for a short time.

One of the most common distracting elements is the feeling of loneliness, even when we are lonely. Just give it the space it needs and watch it: where are you feeling it, what is the feeling?

Feeling angry

Name it impatience, anger, annoyance or even rage it's really all the same at different intensities. Anger is not a very positive emotion, so it appears to be suppressed, but the more we push it down, the more it springs up.

So, allow anger to be present as much as possible. Give it the time and space it requires to unfold.

Feeling of craving

Like anger, there are many different forms of desire. It can be anything from the gentle nagging voice in the back of your mind to a shouting mindset of "I must have it now," for anything, or anyone, for that matter.

Know that the impulse is the subconscious mind trying to flee here and there. But we're never going to have any peace as long as we're running away from that. So, let's just have the urge in the air, but without acting on it.

Integration

Integration is where you implement the peace and understanding that you achieved with the rest of your life during your meditation.

And, what does being conscious and at the moment mean? If you can meditate while sitting on a chair, why not do it while eating your food, drinking a cup of tea, or even walking down the street?

It doesn't mean having your eyes closed down the street though. It simply means having the same sense of being present, concentrated and conscious of the act of walking down the road.

So, instead of dreaming about the holiday you'd love or the new health regime you're about to start, be present and be aware of the physical sensations, sounds, smells and scenery around you.

Stop checking in with how you feel, psychologically, socially, and mentally, when you have a break during your day. It's like creating an image dot-to-dot.

By loading your day with these little points of insight, you can quickly create a larger image together (in this case, calmer, more relaxed, and more focused).

External satisfaction vs. inner peace

One of the issues with this generation is how deeply immersed they are in the pit of technology and how deeply we have incorporated it into our lifestyle.

Some people cannot do anything manually again without the aid of artificial intelligence installed in their devices. A few weeks ago, I was surprised at how a colleague of mine found it difficult to navigate a few blocks without Google Maps.

From technology also, another thing that is eating deeply and voraciously into our society is social media.

Everybody wants to live up to the social media standards, high-quality photos, rich lifestyle, etc.

Below is the story of a client of mine (Miss K.), who was also deep in the social media lifestyle until she spiraled down and later found herself and salvaged her psyche using meditation.

After our sessions, Miss K changed for the better and since then, meditation has been a part of her life. Since we met, she has been practicing it for the last two and a half years.

She has even started training other people for the last four months. But I will get into that a little bit later. Her college career has been eccentric, to say the least.

Miss K started out as pre-med, got halfway through her freshman year in college, before realizing that really wasn't for her. She switched her major about four times before finally landing on international studies and eventually choosing public health.

I believe it took her a long time to figure out what she wanted to do with her life, for a few reasons.

Firstly, Miss K always struggled with self-confidence, and she would set standards for herself so high, that anytime she failed to reach them, or felt she wasn't doing what she was supposed to be doing, instead of finding strength from that situation, she would beat herself up in falter.

Second thing is Miss K's concept of achievement, joy and fulfillment was totally misplaced until lately. We are in a society that supports this notion that we need to depend on outside conditions to be fulfilled within.

This is just a notion drilled through our minds, perhaps because we just couldn't comprehend what joy, achievement, and fulfillment is.

Clearly, at various times, those are separate concepts to varying groups of people. It might be the small stuff like enjoying time with loved ones, or wiggling up on the couch; or passing exams, getting hired for the job you want, meeting the one you intend living your life with.

As all these aspects are wonderful things, we always depend on things that will make us satisfied elsewhere other than ourselves. This concept of external material development has now been exacerbated with the boosts in innovations and also the emergence of the social media.

When we aren't with our smartphones we prob won't really exist any longer, it's almost as if our electronics are becoming other parts of the body without which we can not work.

You're probably reading these through your mobile device for a quick check but if not, you'll most definitely consciously or unconsciously hit one of your computers after dumping this book to search your messages and updates on social media.

Social media: The notion of fake happiness and contentment has been generated through social media. No one really likes to share times of their lives that are negative, no one really likes to publicize their faults or shortcomings.

But internet has made it appear that everybody is constantly productive, always comfortable, always fulfilled. What if we don't have stuff going as we want?

What if we don't attain the certification we desire? What if the individual we were dreaming about living our life with and making them our second half breaks up with us? So we will get the work we would like to have but it has a negative side?

Perhaps our manager rocks, or we've got an awful workmate. Ironically, the idea that brought us internal gratification is now pessimistic outwardly.

What I gradually understand is that our achievement is not only fleeting but our satisfaction is entirely contingent.

We're either happy or content whenever something else makes us feel good and content. We're never really happy for being happy. Here's where Miss K discovered that she'd been going the wrong way.

Back to her story, Miss K’s entire life had been on a one-way path to becoming a doctor. Her family is filled with medical professionals, and at the age of seven, she declared to be just like them.

Of course, her incredible parents let out a huge sigh of relief because they didn't have to convince her to go into medicine as other parents usually do. For a long time, that was what she wanted to do until she started learning more about herself, her passions, and interests.

Suddenly, becoming a doctor was less of what she wanted to do, and more of what she felt obligated to do. Because, in her entire life, she was brainwashed that being a doctor was the only way to success.

Miss K was the obedient type, so she always felt her parents knew what was best for her. So instead of being confident to stand up for herself, she went along with it.

In early college days she was miserable. Was taking classes that she hated, and definitely doing poorly in them. The person she thought she'd spend her life with broke up with her the moment he went to college.

Miss K was still living at home, so it felt like she wasn't getting day-to-day college experience. After years of having a plan and a direction for her life, all of a sudden, she was lost.

And as usual, when you go through hard times or through a break-up, everybody tells you to go out there, do things for yourself, blow off some steam, etc. which she did, Miss K would hang out with friends, would go curl up with a book at a bookstore, she even joined their dance team at school.

Sometimes, she would get a massage. But those were temporary satisfactions. She would still come home and still feel internally dissatisfied with herself.

Social media became the misery of her existence because she saw other people enjoying the things she did not have;

She'd see her friends, ex, and all her classmates posting pictures of their college adventures, their dorm rooms, their new friends, etc. and all those things made her feel like a failure for a couple of reasons:

Firstly, since she was still living at home, her life was pretty much boring so she didn't have anything to share on social media. Miss K did not feel like she was having the conventional college experience.

Secondly, based on her family's legacy, she wasn't meeting the standard of success that had been laid down for her. Her academic performance wasn't doing well for someone who aspired to become a doctor.

But because good grades were the only definition of success she knew, she was stuck in it, and her CGPA and self-esteem failed as a reason.

This usually happens when we have misplaced priorities, we keep feeling bad and beating ourselves up because some things that we probably do not need in the path to our success begin to fail.

So how did she change for the better? Well, she had support. It is funny how self-therapy is almost never done alone.

We are always in need of assistance, a coach, a mentor, a friend to motivate us and most of all, a good listener.

She was able to have a few people who fit into those roles and with time and effort she started meditation and though it took her a very long time to get to a point where she became consistent with meditation, she was able to gain a lot:

Confidence: by creating a consistent reconnection with her inner self, she drove that fear and lack of confidence away.

Suddenly, she was able to stand up for herself and was feeling more confident within herself, to the point that it gave her the courage to eventually switch her major to International Studies, and got rid of the idea that in order to be successful, she had to do something big.

Replacing the positive with the negative We might get the career we wish, but there will still be some bad or something about it, we wouldn't want to cope with it.

Then the whole world becomes pessimistic. Cultivating a connection with her internal self through meditation allowed her to see the positive in any situation regardless of what it was.

Communication: initially or while growing up, Miss K was non-assertive most of the time, but by creating a connection with herself through meditating constantly, she was able to say the things she needed to say, and speak up for herself when the need arose.

Minimizing stress and anxiety: being able to create confidence in herself made her take on life-altering challenges without any worry or fear of failure.

The capacity to love: as corny as it sounds, the more and more she was able to love herself, the more she was also able to love everything around her.

The lesson to learn is that we shouldn't need to depend on outside conditions to make us happy within.

Real success occurs as you take the trouble to focus on you personally each single day - and develop the qualities you would like to see in you professionally; then you can hang on to all the ideals and communicate them in every external circumstances, whether good or bad.

We think these changes happen to all of us as we grow older well no, they always appear because we choose to. We hope as we move out we're going to know how to cook, we're going to work out more when we actually need it. But this is not the truth.

If we decide to eat we'll know how to. If we decide to work out and train, we will learn how to work out then to training. Miss K's inner self-conception did not alter until she decided consciously to alter her inner self-concept.

For me, real success is about being capable of learning so much more about myself with the meditation every day; and it should be used and demonstrate it in any circumstance in which I am put.

Why meditation seems difficult (the noise in our world)

Connecting with the meditation took me quite a time, due to the fact that I wasn't used to the solitude that comes with meditation.

As beings, I believe we are dependent on noise, since it made people feel like we're doing stuffs.

So I'm sitting to meditate and I'd remember about 5 or 10 minutes later that I was missing noise, I wanted that form of compromise.

So I would give up on sleep so I looked for my smartphone or my desktop automatically. What it was telling me was that I had reached a point that I despised quietness.

It showed me just how noisy my life was. Noise isn't just static or cacophony; hum (or noise) is the annoyance you experience with a member of your family or acquaintance.

If it's noisy enough to annoy us, almost anything is disturbance. As I learned that I had come to despise quietness, I got my behavior checked.

I found that without sounds, or vibration, or disturbances of some kind, I couldn't get past a day. I'd wake up then meditate half-heartedly till giving up, as it was getting too intense.

I would immediately reach for my phone for my laptop, and I would play some sound and videos while I was getting ready for school or while I was eating breakfast.

I'd drive to school with the audio on, I'd get to class, I'd be fine; about halfway through the class, I'd zone out thinking about some video I watched or a game I played.

Due to my emotions and worries, there would be much more confusion swirling around me and through me that I would come home feeling irritated, and let that anger out on my relatives not understanding what to do about it.

I will continue my research and feel upset because I did not understand the principles, but that's only because I got background sounds. As the day ends, I actually sit back to meditate, and I would give it up again be as there was far too much happening in my mind.

I got upset as I could not fall asleep but then I was disappointed since I felt like I didn't advance with my practice in meditation.

What it really showed me to create a viable link to my true self was that I would have to learn to love quiet.

To know how to enjoy harmony I have to really use my determination and stick to my routine of meditation. My inner world had to communicate with my outside setting to maintain my affection for the peace that I created internally.

The more I was meditating, the further I began learning how to enjoy solitude emotionally, the further my inner world continued to mirror my outer setting. That was when I was beginning to see all the improvements I needed to see in myself.

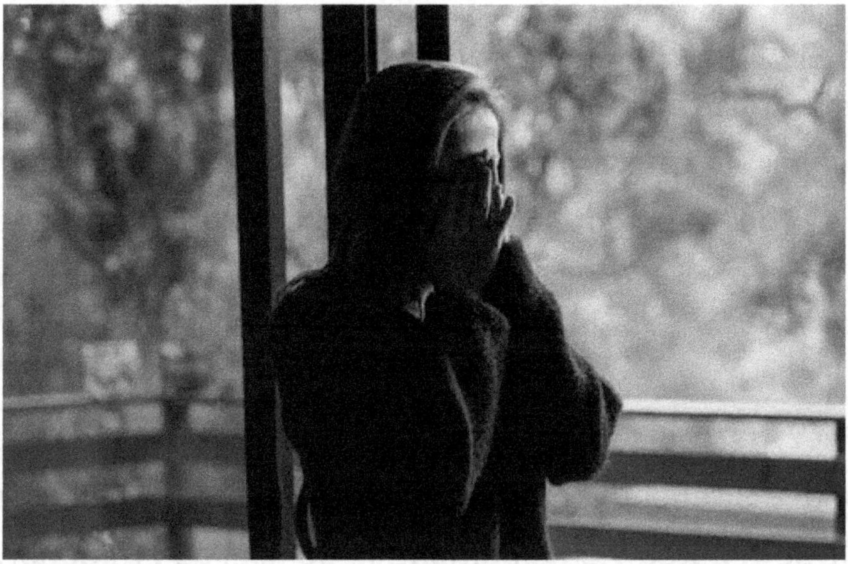

Narcissistic psychopathology is interpreted as a blend of three complex factors:

- A pronounced deficiency in self-esteem and self -cohesion.
- A concerted attempt to balance the shortfall by seeking positive outlets of self-affirmation.
- Seeking self-affirmation whilst not compromising interpersonal weakness.

The shape of interpretation is frequently used to assist the affected person to understand the frequently intense feelings of the therapist about any empathic failure and realize that when being hurt by means of any broken empathic (self-object) bonds, he (the affected person) should regain power and comfort.

The affected person starts off evolved to understand and apprehend perfectly why he might also locate those reputedly small empathic deficits as profoundly as comprehension emerges.

The narcissistic remedy of sufferers is approached from the point of view of Kohut's principle of self-psychology, and the outcomes and issues encountered with this process are described and mentioned.

Narcissistic persona ailment (NPD) is one of the least recognized persona problems.

Although, in a small number of patients diagnosed with depressive disorders or other mood symptoms at a psychiatrist's workplace, the prognosis of narcissistic trends is recorded to be present.

The prevalence of complete-blown NPD inside the psychiatric network varies from 2% to 16% and typically happens in the trendy population at a rate of much less than 1%.

That shape of the disorder is regularly observed in guys who've happened to be guys with almost 50-seventy five percentage of NPD instances.

NPD's principal characteristics are such signature behavior styles could have a substantial terrible impact on a patient's interpersonal relationships and lifestyles.

These patients frequently behave outwardly with an experience of entitlement and superiority, ignore others, and frequently show rude or patronizing attitudes.

However, low and inadequate emotions are at the back of this behavior and are primary to this situation of the character.

At the same time, as many sufferers reap high performance, this condition's symptoms ultimately intrude with both the patient's career and private relationships.

This is due to the fact the patient is frequently unable to get over criticism or rejection, in addition to behaving for others in standard in an empathic way of disrespect.

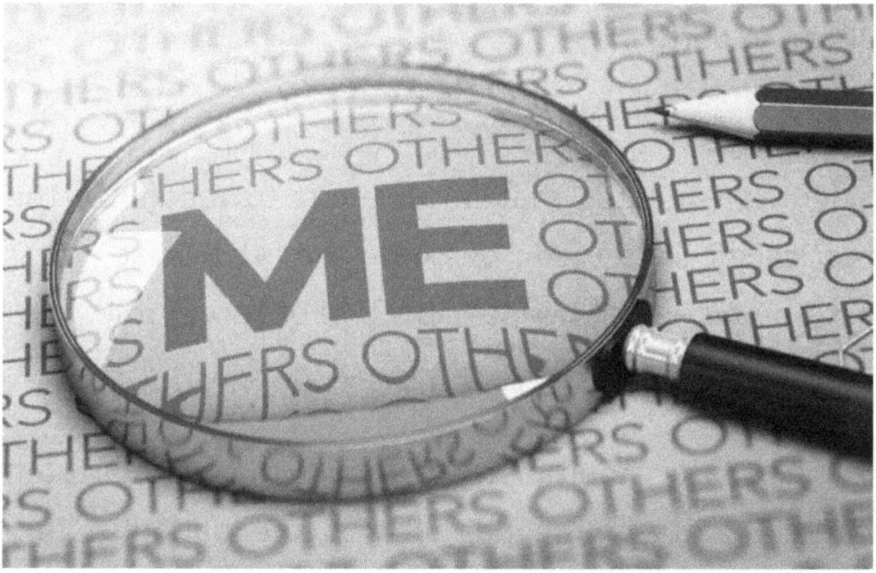

There are numerous hypotheses about the origins of the NPD. For the duration of childhood, there have often been a couple of developmental and maternal elements concerned.

An instance of a developmental factor includes a postulated innate over-sensitive adolescence disposition; parental factors include undue parental affection, lack of realistic parental developmental feedback, insufficient parental care and/or emotional abuse in early life.

Scientist indicates that in an effort to recognize the narcissistic affected person, the therapist must assume an empathic-introspective observer role.

It helps the therapist to recall the complicated internal parts of the patient and the patient's very own subjective parts which he/she revels in.

The affected person can then talk brazenly, and the therapist is confidential about what the patient represses or wards off.

Self-psychology, like object-family members principle, originated from a trial to deal with sufferers who did now not reply to ego-mental remedy, based totally on analysis of psychological defense.

Scientist argues that in improvement, adult narcissistic psychopathology is made from parental lack of empathy.

The toddler does now not expand the ability to alter through refusing to offer good empathic comments within the development of a child at essential stages, and thus the adult vacillates between unreasonable self-overestimation and feelings of inferiority.

Researchers indicates that, underneath regular circumstances, the growing child has critical mental structures: the grandiose-exhibitionist self (usually evolving into self-assertive ambitions) and the idealized parental imago (generally evolving into internalized values and beliefs).

First-area pathology contributes to grandiosity susceptibility, at the same time as latter-area pathology leads to deficits, in which psychopathology is rooted in fixations on patriarchal idealizations.

A system that maintains to conform (thru self-object formation) is the dyad that happens between a baby and his dad and mom.

A self-object in Kohut's theory consists of the developing toddler plus every one of these folks that give the child the potential to preserve self-structure and steadfastness, and a sense of unity and steadfastness.

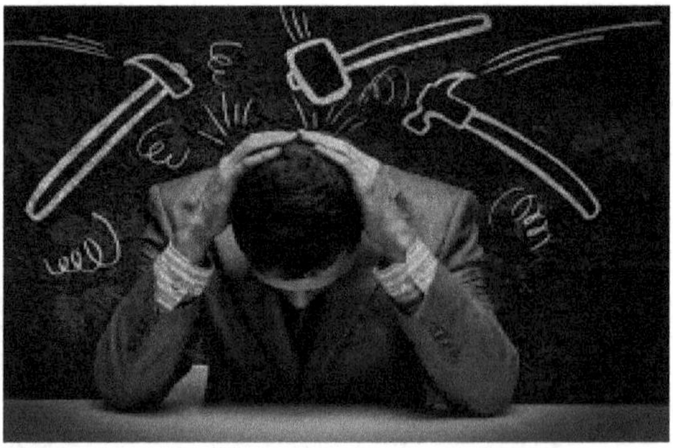

We're self-gadgets because, in line with scientist, the kid is unaware of not being part of himself or herself and of performing roles which the kid will later learn to play on its very own.

A developmental arrest is taking vicinity underneath Kohut's model, and pathological narcissism will emerge while certain self-item desires are not empathically met.

Researcher's describes three reasons for this obvious loss of parental empathy:

1) Terrible verbal exchange among the child and the dad and mom with regards to the disposition of both parties.

2) The parents unable to react to and nurture the infant, which could frequently be because of physical or mental barriers.

3) The kid has a surprisingly high want for self-objects (which parents may not be able to give).

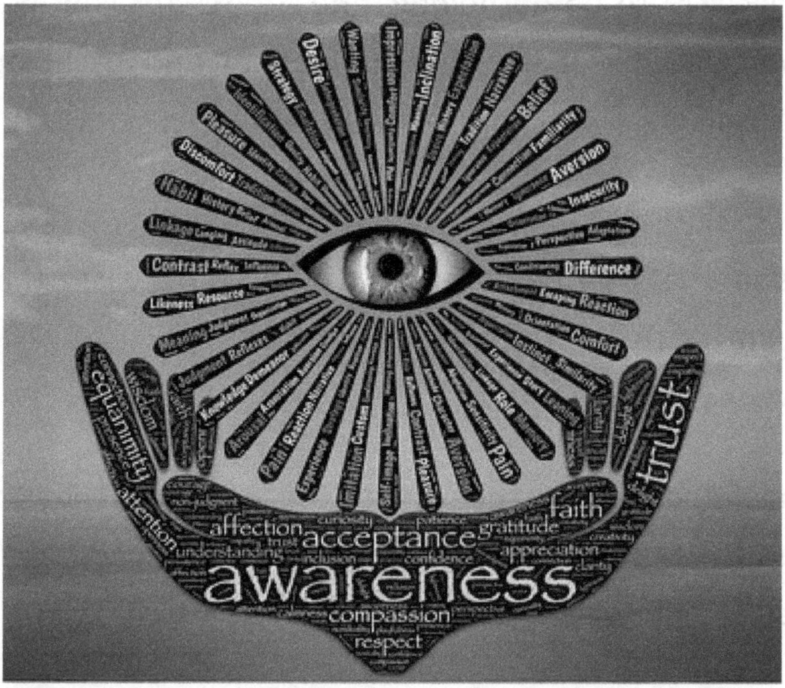

Scientist describes the self as “the centre of the psychological universe” and believes we spend our entire lives looking for how to construct and keep ourselves through the use of things related to our self.

But, in the evaluation of different theorists, Researchers do not take into account this form of narcissism to be pathologic and argues for continuity amongst normal infantile narcissism and pathologic narcissism.

Researchers argues that pathologic narcissism takes ground early with self-parts screwing up.

Whilst those screw-ups arise, those patients look for gratification of missing formative year's self-object desires of their adult lives.

They are also fearful of encountering or repeating, earlier past failures. Therefore, they'll present with an attitude of superiority or haughtiness, reflecting tension they feel over encountering in addition to self -item failures.

This fear can also occur in relationships. Sufferers with NPD may additionally have a history of many failed relationships secondary to sadness that the connection isn't giving them the longed-for adolescence gratification and their lacking self-object desires.

Scientist emphasizes that all of us desire to be ideal, that absolutely everyone does not forget himself in a grandiose way, and that each one's desires and thoughts aren't to start with negative things.

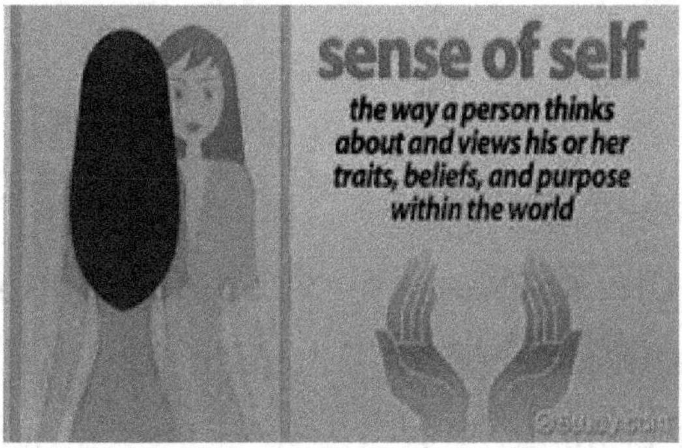

However, with good parenting, those thoughts are gradually lessened through the years (despite the fact that in no way in reality are they destroyed) thru inevitable minor self-object screw-ups or best frustrations.

These minor frustrations are necessary for shaping a child's experience of self; however, they are not psychologically stressful.

Research factors out that it is probably defective to consider parents can (or must) at all times meet the self-object desires of a child as mother and father as they themselves are human and are not with the kid at all times.

Scientist believes those failures are crucial to regulating the innate grandiose delusional thoughts with which we're born because of the fact they require the child to investigate inner mechanisms to self-sooth and keep his or her self, however not being ideal.

Once the self's mechanisms are grounded, the child is based lot less on self-items for appreciation and rises to regulate self-esteem because the child can alter the feeling himself.

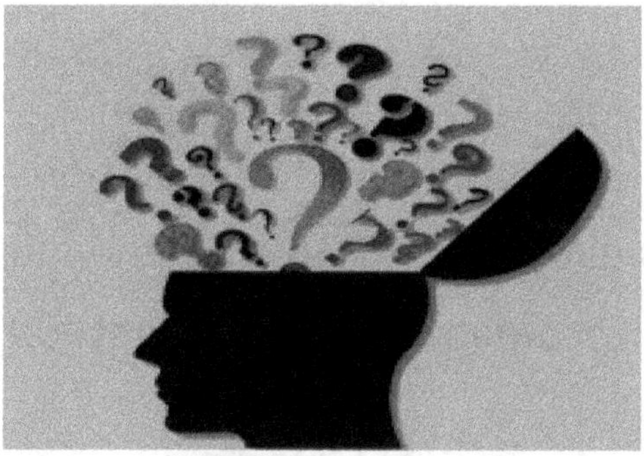

In the narcissistic affected character, self-object desires had been not met sooner or later of one’s youth, and so one's mechanisms in no way develop and he/she will usually make an appearance to others (self-devices) for buttressing self-esteem.

Therefore, the narcissistic person may be very sensitive to any criticism or obvious rejection.

Practice elements.

Mother and father usually meet self-item desires of a toddler in big component through strategies:

The parent displays back to the child the emotions and mind that the child is experiencing to offer the kid an enjoyment of being examined and understood (mirroring transference).

And the situation makes the kid desire to view the discernment as his or her protector and feel a sense of energy and luxury from doing so (idealizing transference).

Inside the path of remedy with a narcissistic affected individual, those self-object needs can emerge and are referred to as self-object transferences.

The two transferences that most customarily surface in remedy are the mirroring and idealizing transferences.

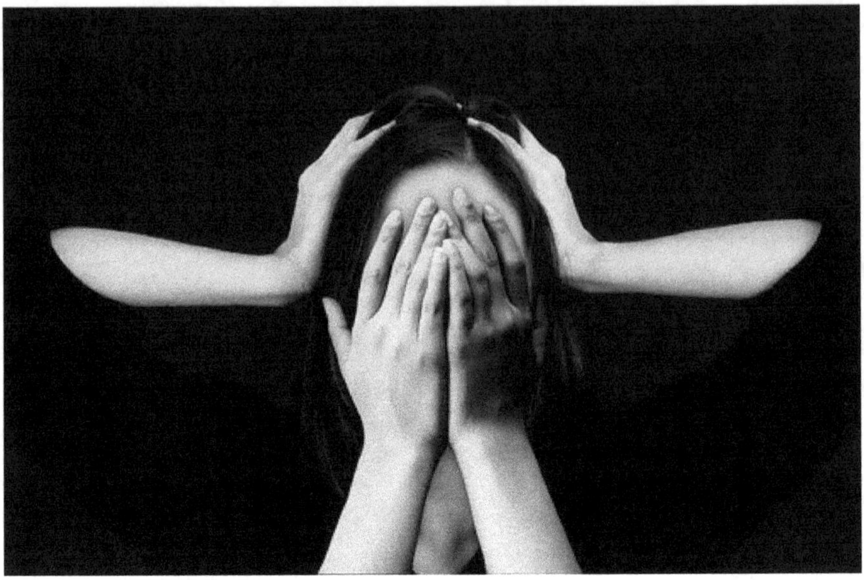

Your non-public internal communication can both be an effective stepping stone or a high impediment to reaching your goals.

In case you continuously make bad predictions like, "I am going to mess up," otherwise you name yourself names, your self-talk will rob you of intellectual power.

Your thoughts have an effect on the way you experience things and the way you behave. The way you think has the electricity to turn out to be a self-satisfying prophecy.

Wondering, "I will in no way get this procedure" might also motivate you to sense discouraged as you walk into an interview.

Consequently, you may slump your shoulders, stare on the ground, make a terrible first impact—and inadvertently sabotage your probabilities of fulfilment.

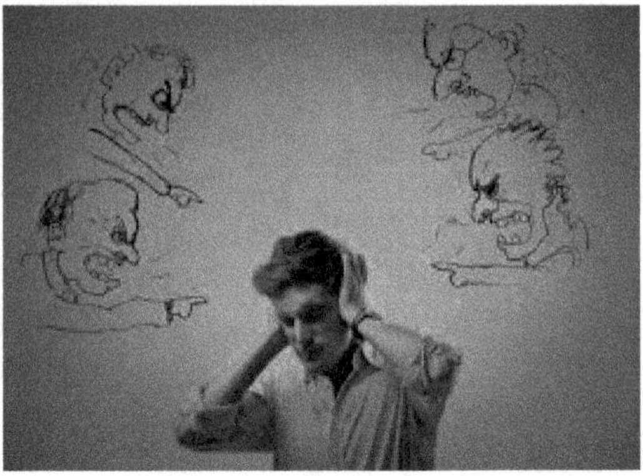

From most of the many sporting activities that we use in treatment to help human beings alternate the manner they anticipate, proper here are seven approaches to tame your internal critic:

1. Take note of your thoughts.

You're so used to listening to your very own narration that it is very simple to become oblivious to the messages you are sending yourself.

Start paying good interest to your mind, and you may find out that you call yourself names or communicate yourself out of doing things which might be difficult. It's far from prediction that you have centered in your mind thousands of things daily.

It virtually is thousands of possibilities to both build yourself up or tear yourself down. Getting to know to understand your notion styles is fundamental to knowing how your questioning affects your lifestyles.

2. Trade the channel.

Even as problem-fixing is useful, ruminating is unfavorable.

At the same time as you maintain replaying a mistake you made to your head over and over once more otherwise you can't forestall considering a few awful factors that passed off, you will drag yourself down.

The great manner of trading the channel is by means of getting lively. Discover an interest which will, in brief, distract you from the negative tapes gambling for your head.

Pass for a stroll, call a chum to talk about one-of-a-kind trouble or address an assignment you have been casting off. But refuse to sit down and deal with your mind till it beats you up.

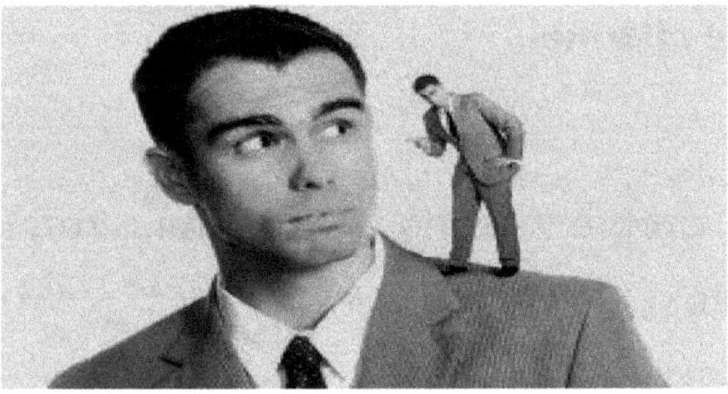

3. Have examined the proof.

Your mind isn't continuously going to be genuine. In fact, it will often exaggeratedly terribly. It is crucial to study the situation forehand than you believe your thoughts.

In case you assume, "I'm just going to embarrass myself when I make that presentation" pause for a minute.

Take out a chunk of paper and write down all the evidence that shows you are going to fail.

Then, list all of the evidences which propose you aren't going to fail. Searching at the evidence on every facet permits you to have a look at the situation a hint extra rationally and much less emotionally.

Reminding yourself that your mind is not a hundred percentage on-point can offer you a lift in self-assurance.

4. Update exaggeratedly horrible thoughts with practical statements.

Even as you understand that your terrible thoughts aren't truly right, strive to change the one's statements with something more practical.

If you think, "I'll in no way get a raise" a fantastic replacement assertion is probably, "If I go tough I continue investing in myself, I may get a raise ultimately."

You do not need to increase unrealistically in exquisite statements; overconfidence may be nearly as poor as excessive self-doubt.

However, a balanced, practical outlook is fundamental to becoming mentally stronger.

Don't forget how terrible it is in case your mind has been real.

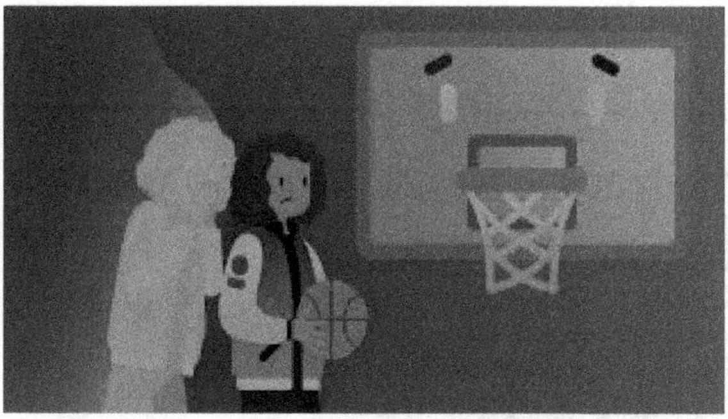

It's far tempting to examine a misstep becoming an utter catastrophe, but often the worst-case situation is not as awful as we worry.

If you predict you will get rejected for a system, ask yourself how horrible ought to that truly be? Rejection stings, but it's no longer the give up of the arena. Reminding yourself that you may.

Tell yourself what recommendation you need to provide a relative. It's far regularly less difficult for others to be extra compassionate to you than you are to yourself.

For example, even as for falling in a mistake, you would possibly name yourself an idiot, it is unlikely you would do this to a cherished one.

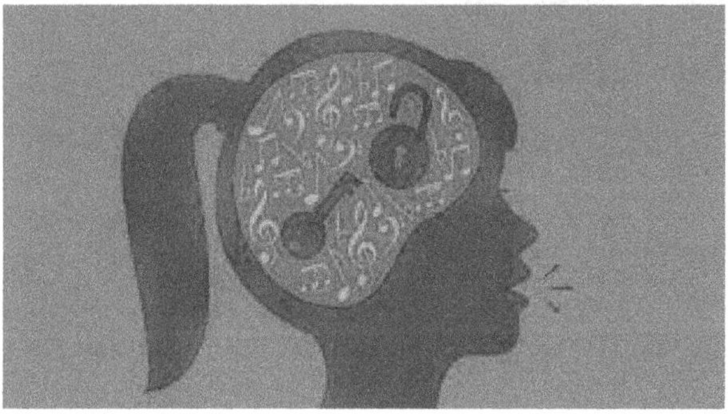

Whilst you are coping with tough times or doubting your capability to be successful, ask yourself, "What would I do to a chum who this happened to or if my wife fell into this or children?"

Self-development, coupled with self-recognition.

There may be a difference among pronouncing, but they are similar. Self-development is when you put efforts in advancing your mind and, body.

Self-recognition is knowing, understanding and ability to maintain your mind and body giving each its rights.

Don't forget the shortcomings as they make a contribution to exchange within the destiny for what they are proper now.

Although it sounds a chunk counterintuitive, you may do each at the identical time: you might agree that you're feeling hectic about an upcoming presentation at work while also making a decision to broaden your competencies in public talking.

Permit for who you're proper now at the same time as investing in making yourself a fair higher version down the street.

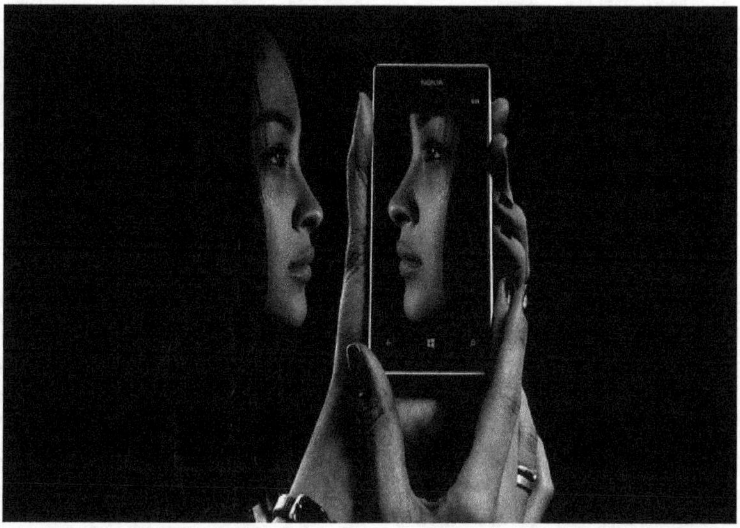

The self is taken into consideration to be the core of the mental world of a person in self-psychology.

If the developmental surroundings of an individual (adult or young) are sufficient, a wholesome experience of the “self” will commonly develop, and the person will normally be able to keep stable patterns at some point of life, self-regulating and self-soothing.

If individuals are not able to broaden a healthful feel of the “self”, they'll be probable to depend upon others to satisfy their wishes.

Those others are self-objects (because they are out of doors of themselves). In line with Khoum, self-items are like a herbal a part of the development system.

Children require self-gadgets because they're not able to fulfil all their own needs.

However, self-items are internalized inside the course of healthful improvement as individuals expand the capability to meet their personal desires without counting on external others.

Often vast for self-psychology is the role of transference. The switch is understood in psychoanalysis as the phase in which someone in remedy transfers feelings and dreams from youth to a brand new item (typically the analyst).

Researchers have proposed three particular styles of transfers that constitute unmet self-object desires:

Mirroring: others act as a replicate on this type of shifting that represents a feeling.

Just as humans use a mirror to check their look, transference mirroring consists of using other human beings' maintaining and encouraging reactions to look nice inside themselves.

Idealizing:

Scientist believed that human beings want people to cause them to experience calm and comfortable moments.

Another instance of this could be visible in youngsters who run after falling or doing a bad deed run to others for refuge.

The opposite person is idealized or thought as someone who's calm and calming when he isn't viable to provide it on their personal.

Twin ship/alter Ego:

Researchers advised that people have to behave like others. Children, as an instance, need to be near their dad and mom who'll make children-like actions with them.

An infant will become more able to tolerate variations when he notices similar infant-like behavior from the parent.

Self-Image.

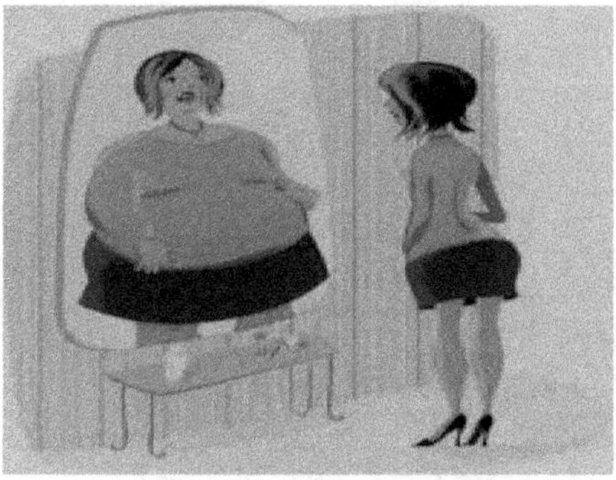

The way we see ourselves is the self-image. Self-image includes what we recognize visually about ourselves (e.g. brown hair, blue eyes, tall), our social roles (e.g. wife, uncle, gardener), and our character traits (e.g. friendly, intense, kind).

Self-image does not constantly correspond to reality. Many humans have a distorted view of 1 or extra parts in their traits.

Such distorted perspectives can be both superb and negative, and a person may also have an extra high-quality view of some factors of the self and a greater poor view of others.

Self-focus.

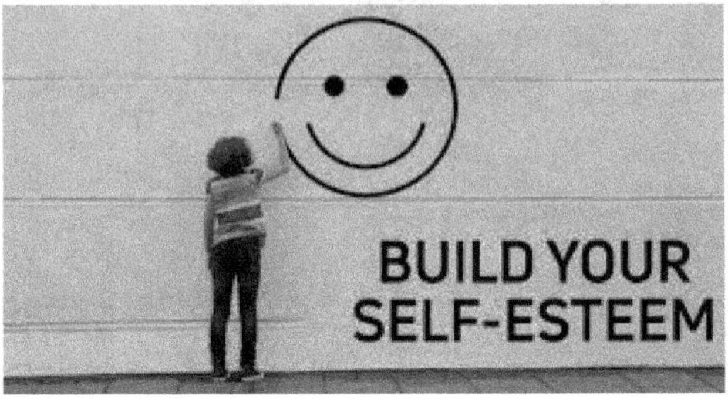

The importance we placed on ourselves is character levels rely upon how we measure ourselves. Such judgments encompass our own studies with others as well as the reactions of others to us.

If we compete with others and locate that we're better at something than others and/or that human beings respond undoubtedly to what we're doing.

On the other hand, our declines whilst we equate ourselves with others and find that we aren't at the top in a given location and people respond negatively to what we do.

In a few ways ("I am an awesome professional") we will have experts even as at the same time you will be poor in other things ("I am now not properly-preferred").

Ideal self.

The perfect or ideal self is what we want to be, our highest dreams of what we want ourselves to be. Regularly there may be a distinction between the self-image of one and the ideal-self of individuals.

This incongruity could have a bad impact on one's self -image as well as ideal-self. Compatibility among the self-picture and the perfect-self requires a truthful amount of variant between the 2.

Even though reaching best congruence is tough, if not impossible, extra congruence will permit for self-actualization.

Incongruence among self-image and the perfect-self is certain, a disparity takes place among one's self and one's experiences, resulting in internal war (or cognitive dissonance) that forestalls self-actualization.

Self-idea; self-idea formation is starting to increase in the early formative years. Though, the maximum improvement is generated with the aid of self-idea among early formative years and adolescence.

Children begin to distinguish from others by their growing to around age two. Children take into account that they may be separate and specific selves with the aid of their growing to around three to four.

At this level, the self-picture of a baby is basically descriptive, predominantly based totally on bodily or concrete info. Although children are steadily listening to their abilities, and by getting to the age of 6, children can express what they need and desire.

Between a long term of seven and eleven, children start to make social comparisons and remember how they’re perceived by way of others.

At this level, youngsters' descriptions of themselves end up more in summary.

They start to describe themselves in terms of capabilities and no longer simply concrete info, and they understand that their traits exist on a continuum.

As an instance, an infant at this stage will begin to see himself as more athletic than some and less athletic than others, instead of sincerely athletic or not athletic. At this point, the right self and self-photography start to develop.

Early life is a key length for self-idea. The self-idea hooked up at some point of youth is generally the basis for the self-idea for the rest of one's life.

In the course of the adolescent years, humans experiment with extraordinary roles, personas, and selves. For teenagers, self-concept is motivated by way of achievement in areas they price, and the responses of others valued to them.

Success and approval can make a contribution to greater and a more potent self-idea into adulthood.

The diverse Self-idea.

We all hold several various ideas about ourselves. A number of those thoughts may also be loosely associated, and some may additionally even be contradictory.

These contradictions do not create trouble for us, however, due to the fact we're aware of just a few of our self-concept at any given point in time we think they create it.

Self-concept is made of more than one self-schemas: man or woman concepts of a selected issue of the self.

The idea of self-schema is useful when thinking about self-concept as it explains how we will have a specific, nicely-rounded self-schema about one issue of the self even as missing a concept about every other issue.

As an instance, one person may see herself as prepared and conscientious, a second person may also see himself as disorganized and scatter-brained, and a third individual may additionally have no opinion in anyway whether or not she is organized or disorganized.

Cognitive and Motivational Roots.

The improvement of self-schema and the larger self-idea has cognitive and motivational roots.

We generally tend to set records about the self very well than information about other matters.

At the equal time, consistent with the self-notion idea, self-understanding is acquired in plenty the equal manner as we accumulate knowledge about others.

We have a look at our behaviors and draw conclusions about who we are from what we note.

Even as people are prompted to are trying to find out this self-know-how, they're selective within the records to which they pay interest

Malleable Self-concept.

Our capacity to call up positive self-schemas even as ignoring others makes our self-concepts malleable.

In a given moment, our self-concept is depending on the social situations in which we discover ourselves and the remarks we receive from the surroundings.

In some instances, this malleability method that makes certain elements of the self can be especially salient.

As an example, a 14-year-old can also grow to be specifically aware of her youth whilst she is with a group of aged adults.

If the identical 14-yr-vintage became in a group of other younger people, she might be a lot much less likely to think about her age.

Self-idea can be manipulated by asking people to keep in mind instances once they behaved in a certain way.

If requested to remember instances once they worked hard, people are usually able to accomplish that; if requested to keep in mind instances when they have been lazy, individuals are also commonly capable of achieving this.

Many human beings can take into account times of both of these opposing traits, but people will generally perceive themselves as one or the other (and act according to that perception) depending on which one is delivered to mind.

On this manner, self-idea may be altered and changed.

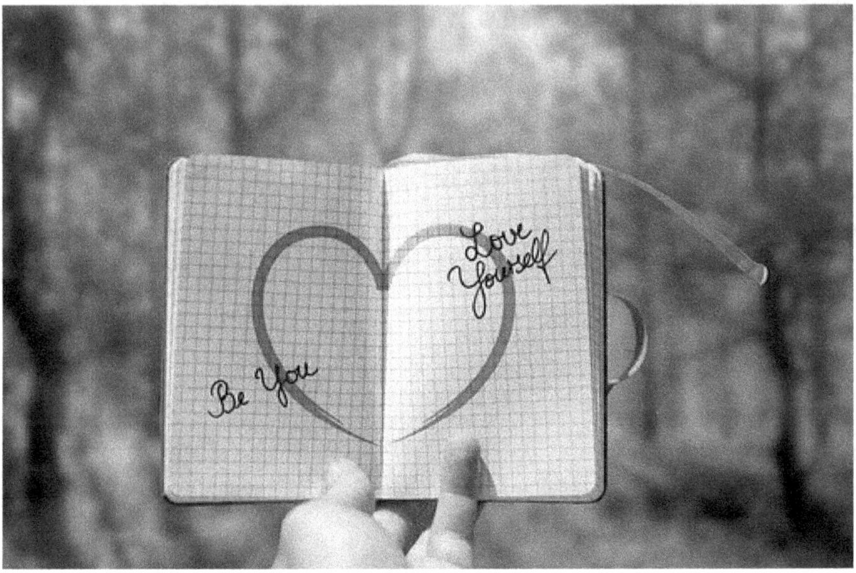

Ranges of Cognitive improvement.

It is believed that as youngsters grow and their brains broaden, they pass thru about four distinct tiers which can be characterized with the aid of differences in idea processing.

In a research carried out, researchers cautiously located kids and supplied them with issues to resolve that were related to item permanence, reversibility, deductive reasoning, transitivity, and assimilation (defined underneath).

Each degree builds upon understanding found out in the previous level. Piaget's four ranges correspond with the age of the kids and are the ***sensorimotor, preoperational, concrete operational, and formal operational stages***.

Sensorimotor degree.

The sensorimotor degree happens from start to age two. It's characterized via the concept that infants "think" with the aid of manipulating the sector round them.

This is executed by using all five senses: seeing, listening to, touching, tasting, and smelling. Kids figure out methods to exhibit responses via “doing”, such as pulling a lever on a song to listen a sound, placing a block in a bucket and pulling it out, or throwing an object to see what occurs.

Among five and eight months antique, the kid develops item permanence, that's the understanding that even though something is clearly wrong, it still exists.

For instance, a child learns that even though his mother leaves the room, she has now not ceased to exist; in addition, a ball does now not disappear due to the fact a bucket is positioned in front of it.

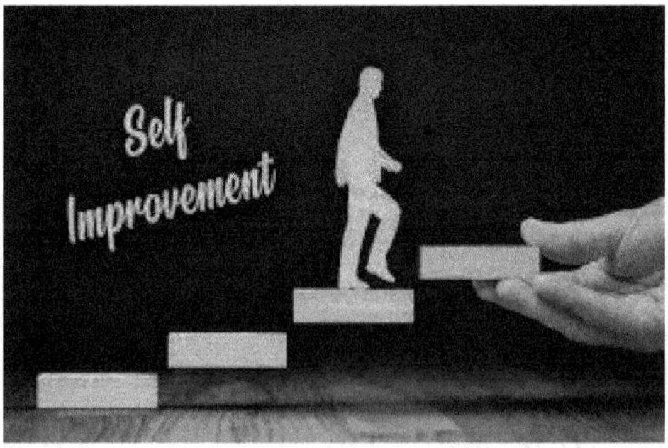

By means of the senses of this stage, kids are able to engage in what Piaget termed deferred imitation.

This includes the capability to breed or repeat a previously-witnessed motion afterwards; instead of copying it proper away, the child is able to produce a mental illustration of it and repeat the conduct in a while.

By way of 24 months, babies are able to imitate behaviors after a delay of up to 3 months.

Preoperational level.

The preoperational level takes place from age 2 to age 7. For the duration of this degree; youngsters can use symbols to represent phrases, pictures, and ideas that is why kids on this level have interaction in faux play.

A baby's hands might turn out to be aircraft wings as she zooms across the room, or a child with a stick may turn out to be a courageous knight with a sword.

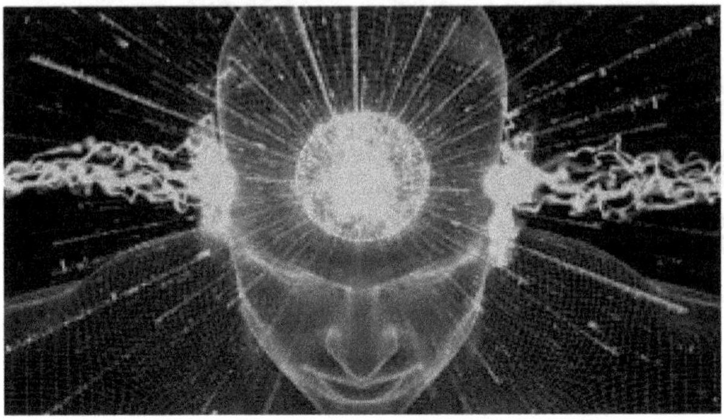

Language improvement and intuitive play starts at some point at this stage. Logical wondering continues to be now no more present, yet they cannot rationalize or understand more complicated thoughts.

Children at this level are very selfish, that means their consciousness is on themselves and the way actions will impact them, instead of others.

They're no longer capable of taking at the attitude of others, and that they suppose that everybody sees, thinks, and feels just like they do.

Concrete Operational degree.

The concrete operational degree happens from age seven to age eleven. It’s characterized with the aid of the idea that youngsters' reasoning becomes focused and logical.

Children reveal logical expertise of conservation principles, the capacity to understand that key objects of a substance do not trade at the same time as their physical look and may be altered.

For example, a child who is familiar with the principles of conservation will apprehend that equal quantity of liquid would take up same surface-are despite the size of the container wherein they may be poured.

Formal Operational.

The formal operational level takes place from age 11 to adulthood. It's far characterized by means of the concept that youngsters expand in the capability to assume and summarize.

This allows youngsters to interact within the trouble-fixing technique of growing speculation and reasoning their manner to potential solutions. Children can think about abstract ideas and feature the potential to combine diverse ideas to create new ones.

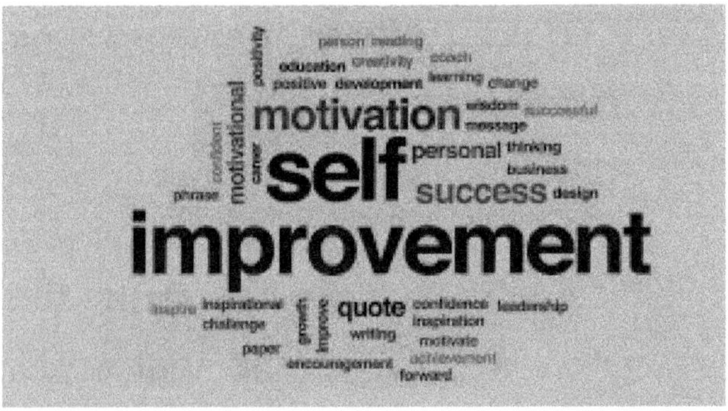

By end of this stage, kids have advanced logical and systematic questioning, kids are able to possess deductive reasoning, and can create hypothetical ideas to explain diverse standards.

Beyond Formal Operational notion.

As with other principal participants of theories of improvement, several of Piaget's thoughts were challenged by way of later research.

In post formal thinking, decisions are made based on conditions and circumstances, and common sense is integrated with emotion as adults broaden concepts that depend upon contexts.

One manner that we are able to see the distinction among an adult in post formal thought and an adolescent informal operations is in terms of how they cope with emotionally charged problems.

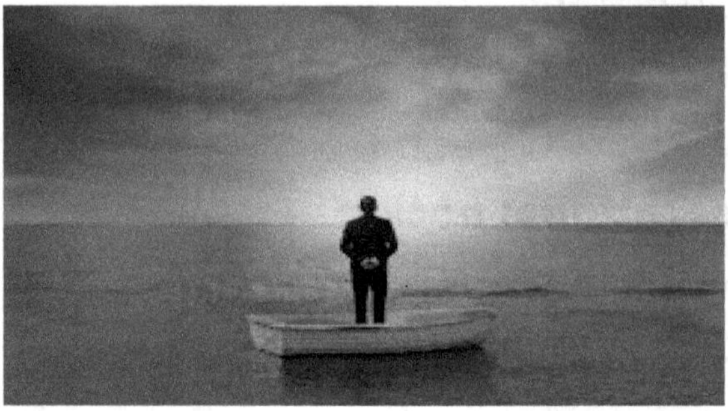

Plainly as soon as we reach adulthood, our problem-fixing competencies change: as we strive to remedy issues, we generally tend to think more deeply about many regions of our lives, together with relationships, work, politics etc.

Because of this, post formal thinkers are capable of drawing on past studies to help them remedy new problems. Problem-solving techniques, the use of post formal idea range relying on the state of affairs.

Adults can recognize, for example, that what appears to be a great solution to a disagreement with a co-worker might not be the best solution for a disagreement with a romantic partner.

Attachments idea.

Attachment theory describes the dynamics of lengthy -term social relationships between human beings.

Attachment in toddlers is mainly a system of proximity-in-search to an identified attachment discern in situations of perceived misery or alarm for the reason of survival.

In other phrases, infants broaden attachment to their caregivers—upon whom they're established—as a way of survival.

Self-idea vs. Self-Efficacy

Self-idea is a greater complex assemble than self-efficacy.

Even as self-efficacy refers to a man or woman's judgments in their own abilities, self-concept is greater well-known and consists of each cognitive (mind related) and affective (emotions related) judgments about oneself.

Self-concept vs. Self-cognizance

Self-awareness additionally impacts self-idea. It is the trait that portrays consciousness of one's own thoughts, emotions, behaviors, and trait.

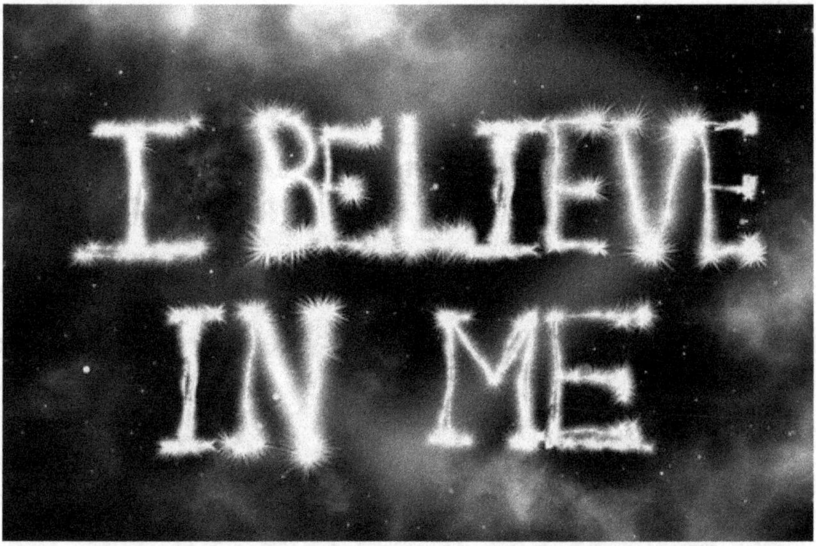

Self-concept protection refers to how humans hold or decorate their feel of self.

It's far noticeably after individuals reaches adulthood. However, it is able to and does trade primarily based on the person’s experiences.

The concept of self-idea safety states that we do not without a doubt sit down and watch for our self-idea to boom: we take a lively function in shaping our self-idea at every age (whether or not we're aware of this).

Self-idea readability and Self-idea Differentiation

Self-concept clarity (SCC) refers to how clear, assured, and constantan character's definitions of oneself are.

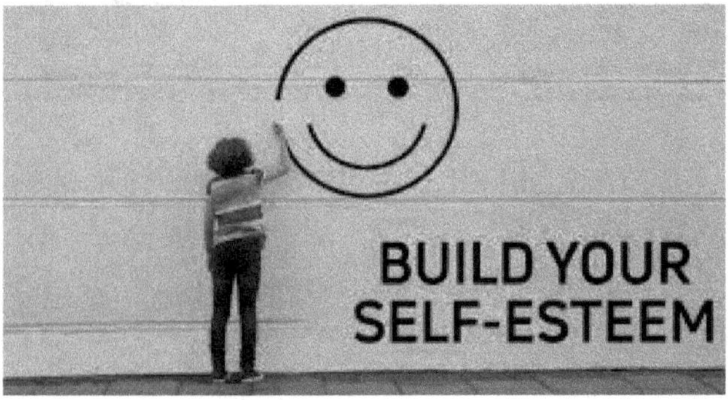

Self-idea differentiation (SCD) refers to how an individual’s self-example may vary for the duration of contexts or social roles (e.g., self as an accomplice, self as a determined worker, and self as a pupil).

SCC and SCD are heat subjects in psychology for the purposes that they have an effect on belief styles and behavior.

Better SCC indicates a more impregnable and stronger self-concept, even as low SCC suggests that an individual is doubtful or vague about who they in reality are.

SCD; not as having a high SCD can be viewed as an awful aspect, but it is able also to be a powerful coping mechanism for succeeding inside the modern world wherein humans have many exclusive roles.

If SCD were very excessive, it would recommend that the man or woman does no longer have a sturdy self-idea and "wears a specific mask" for each of their roles.

A completely low degree of SCD may moreover endorse that the man or woman is authentically "them" for the duration of all in their roles—although it may additionally mean that he cannot effectively transfer from one characteristic to every other.

Basically, folks who differentiate their roles slightly; however, hold a clear picture of themselves, can also achieve success most at locating balance in their identity and picture.

The components and factors of the Self-concept model.

There is the first-rate mind about what self-concept consists of, and the manner it needs to be defined; but, there are some traits and dimensions that apply to the easy, agreed-upon conceptualization of self-concept.

Characteristics of Self-idea

As a brief evaluation, self-idea is the perspective we think we ourselves are. Every human being has a totally specific self-idea, specific from the self-idea of others. Below are some characteristics of self-idea;

- Shows uniquely with everyone.
- Varies from very superb to very bad.
- Includes emotional, intellectual, and practical dimensions.
- Modifications with the context.
- Adjustments over time.

- Have an effect on the character's life.

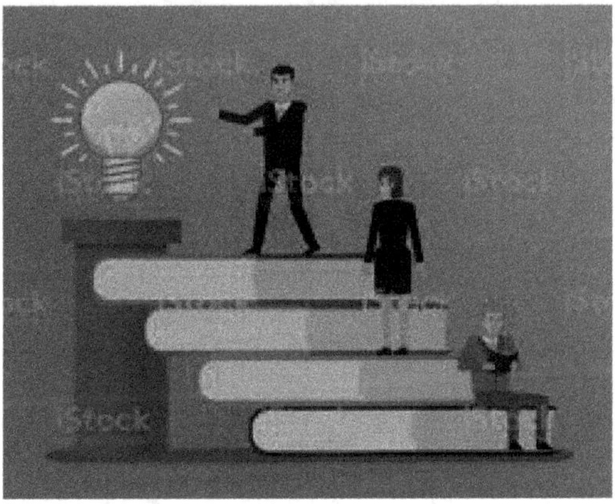

Self-idea in centre early life.

At some stage in centre early life (about 7 to 11 years), kids are starting to broaden a sense of their social selves and figuring out how they suit in with anyone else.

They reference social organizations and make social comparisons greater regularly, and start to not forget how others see them.

The improvement of Self-concept in formative years

Young people are in the period whereby the improvement of their self-idea genuinely explodes.

That is the degree in which people (about age 12-18) play with their sense of self, inclusive of a time once they check with their identity, evaluate themselves with others, and increase the premise of a self-idea that may live with them the rest in their life.

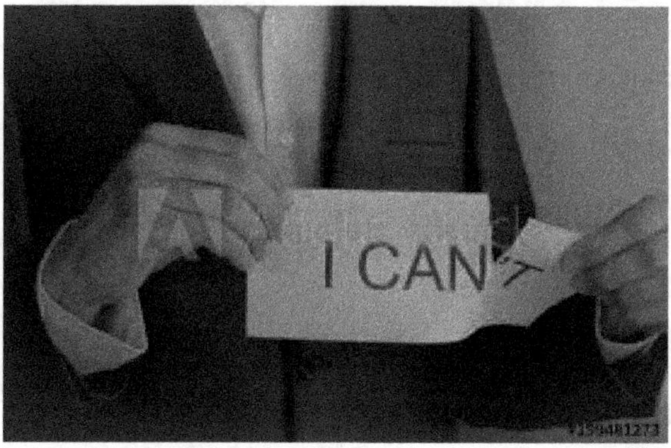

For the duration of this period, younger people are liable to extra self-awareness, and susceptibility to the have an impact on their buddies and chemical changes taking place within the mind.

They experience extra freedom and independence, have interaction in increasingly more competitive sports activities, observe themselves with their peers, and might cost (even over-cost) the angle of others.

In childhood, there are critical elements that have an effect on self-concept:

- Success in areas wherein the achievement of the adolescent desire.

- Approval from enormous people within the adolescent's life.

Examples of Self-concept

You can have a superb deal knowing what self-concept is but these examples can help deliver a cause of it more.

Self-requirements are not frequently all powerful or all bad; someone may also moreover have every fantastic and a few terrible self-ideas in distinctive aspects.

A husband who taught of himself as a very wonderful and caring father but sees his physical self as out-of-form and dangerous or a Scholar who expects themselves as an extremely good personnel but then sees himself as struggling academically.

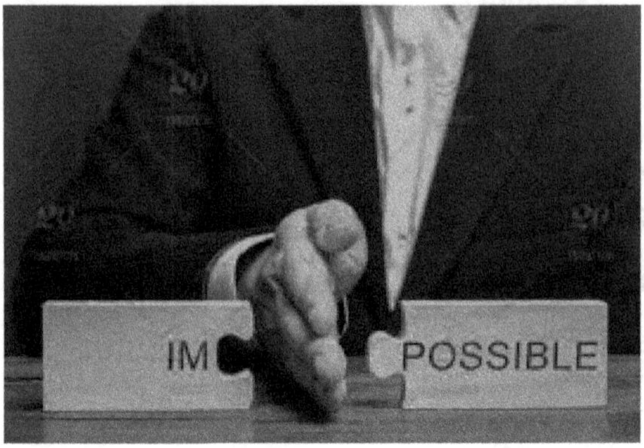

Self-concept in advertising and marketing and how it impacts purchaser's conduct

It'll likely receive a surprise from you that the idea of self-concept has made its way into advertising regardless of the whole lot disused above

Manufacturers and groups can benefit from concentration on superb suitable identities. In reality, it's makes the idea of favor and consumerism.

Our self-idea affects our wants and needs, and also can shape our conduct. Whether or no longer it is authentic or not, we generally tend to believe that our purchases will help set up our identity. There is a cause of why people purchase clothing, automobiles, and lots more than others

Self-idea Attachment

Self-idea attachment refers to the attachment we shape to a product as it impacts identity. As an instance, a person who loves their Patagonia jacket very much would also keep in mind that it is just casual wear.

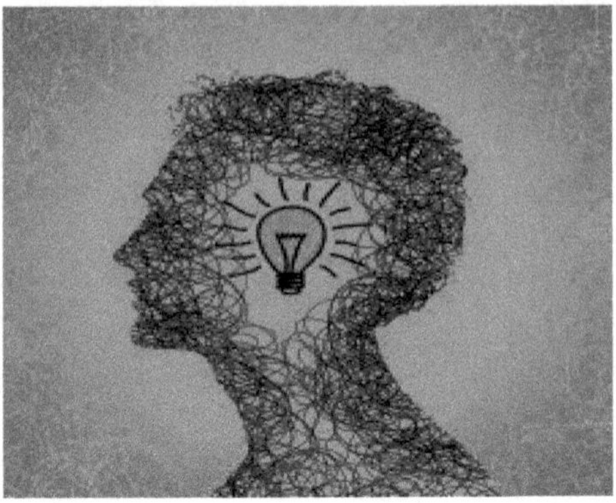

Because of this, this jacket has a strong self-concept attachment, in addition to its motive of imparting warm temperature.

How Does Self-idea have an impact on Interpersonal, verbal exchange?

Don't forget a cycle in which we expand, preserve, and revise our self-concept: we have an idea of who we're, and we act according to that self-concept.

Consequently, they shape the concept of who we're, and self-concept reacts in accordance with the idea of who we are, for that reason we need to be impacting our best concept of who we are.

This remark loop continues to shape us, and interpersonal communication plays a massive function here.

Our self-concept drives our motivations, strategies, and reviews with talking with others.

As an example, if you see yourself as someone who's usually always correct (or who must always be on point), you could flare up in speaking with others whilst disagreements get up.

If that need is determined thru the popularity of aggression, you could use hostility, assertiveness, and argumentativeness to attack the self-ideas of the people you're debating instead of discussing their positions.

Self-idea and educational success

Self-idea and educational achievement is likewise a superb feedback loop, as actions beget comparable moves and identification to suit.

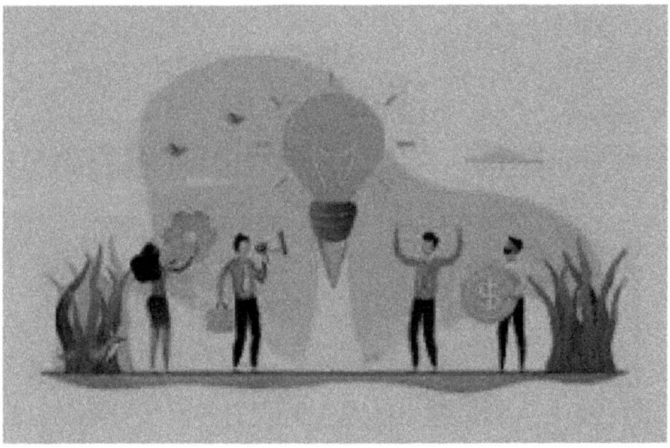

Self-concept and academic success

Self-idea and academic fulfilment is also a nice comments loop, as improvements beget similar moves and identification of being healthy academically.

Its determined that students with more first-class academic self-idea performed greater academic success in the subsequent year.

Later research confirmed the relationship with some of them; however, indicated that fulfilment affects self-idea greater than self-idea inherently impacts success fulfilment.

Self-concept and career improvement

Self-idea develops at a few degrees within the lifespan and at some stage in any profession. The primary degree is marked via the improvement of one's basic self-idea.

In the second degree, capable human beings check and attempt new instructions, reports, and jobs. Degree three sees people setting up their career and constructing their skills, probable starting in a get entry to-diploma function.

In the fourth degree, people interact in a non-preventive control and adjustment setting to both their self-idea and their career.

Ultimately, the 5th level is characterized through a way of reduced output and arrangements for retirement, activities which can have a large effect on one's self-concept.

Way of life and Self-idea

Unsurprisingly, way of life may additionally have a large impact on self-idea. For instance, how kids are handled in early formative years affects how their feelings of “self” develop.

Many dads and moms might be more concerned with feelings and enjoy the desires of their children, whilst others may be greater accompanying and controlling in their infant’s behavior, demanding their needs in the region of pleasing their desires.

Further research additionally indicated that East Asian cultures are extra accepting of contradictory ideals of the self; this suggests that one’s self-concept in those cultures can be more flexible than, say, American region.

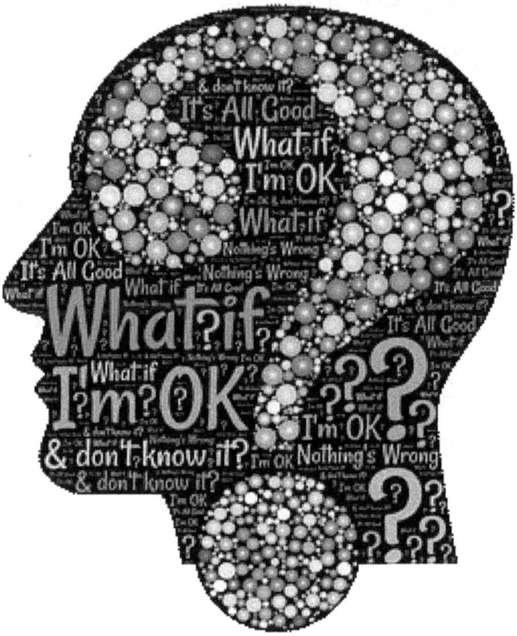

Self-file biasing makes measuring self-concept hard. One's self-concept does not continuously align with "truth" or with how others view a person.

However, there are though a few equipment’s that can bring diplomacy to self-idea.

If you are interested in the usage of a self-concept degree for studies assessment, look first at the development of the tool, the definition it's based on, and the scale it measures.

It’s critical that you pick a tool that aligns with the idea of self-idea that your studies make use of.

The Interview

This is going to be like a test carried out on the students. This act is tremendous as students to get to recognize their pals.

Break them into pairs, and make certain each student is paired with someone they don't thoroughly flow with.

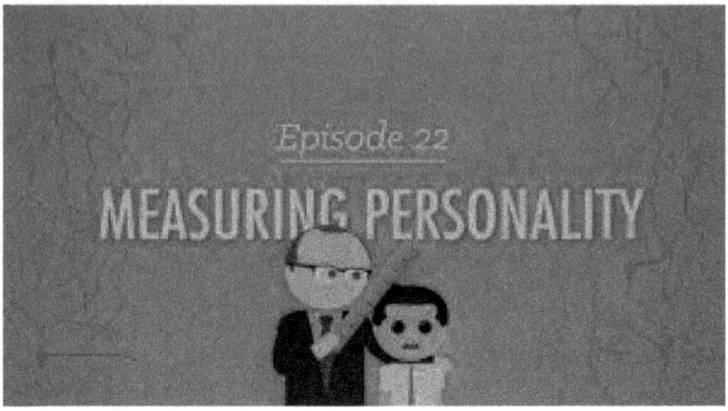

Give them 10 minutes to interview every different unit you've made them to, with funny questions like

"ought to you as an alternative stay on a boat or on an island?" or "what's your favoured problem at this school?"

Whilst all the interviews were finished, have each pair come to the front of the class and introduce their companion to the alternative kids.

The magazine

Journals may be beneficial in masses of approaches, as getting a magazine lets in you to self-test.

Help your college students boom their feel of self via assigning magazine entries that they maintain in a single notebook all year.

Inform your college students that they can put anything they need in their journal they are able to write a poem, describe a dream that they had, write about what they choose for, some element they are happy about, something they are sad about, and so on.

And they need to make at least three entries (or however much you make a decision which is suitable) in keeping with it weekly. Confirm to be certain they've at least three dated entries per week

Rating trends

This hobby is wonderful for older students with writing skills. Have the scholars rip a piece of paper into ten strips and write a phrase or phrase on every strip that they think describes them.

Inform them that no individual will see the things they write down, so they may be completely sincere.

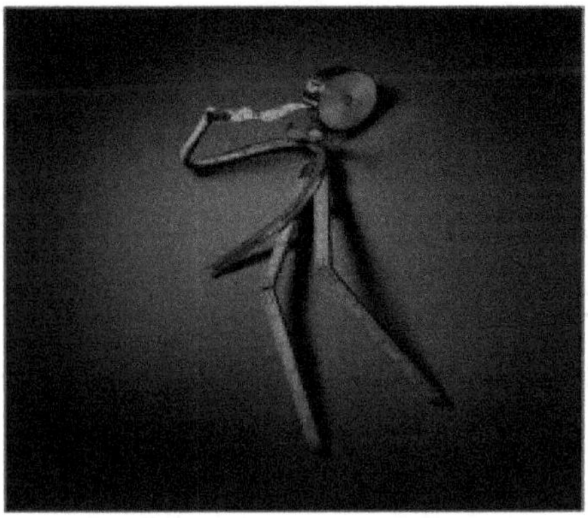

Once the students have written down their ten entries, have them arrange them in order from those they maximum like about themselves to those they least like about themselves.

Thumbprints

This pastime calls for an ink pad and the willingness to get a chunk messy!

Have every of your college students place his or her thumb at the inkpad after which on a chunk of paper to get a thumbprint.

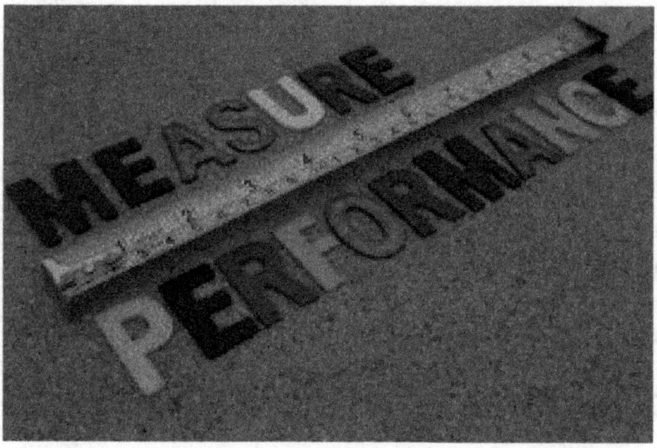

Display them the five main fingerprint patterns and get them to pick out their print type.

Give an explanation for how fingerprints are particular—both across their hands and from person to person.

Subsequently, have each pupil create an animal out of their thumbprint.

Bonus elements if the animal is one, the animal the student feels represents her or him! Inspire them to write this down in their journal, or to add the thumbprint drawing to their mag.

Create a "Me" enterprise

This hobby may be especially amusing for the drama-loving college students. Tell them that they're going to make a two or three-minute business enterprise.

The economy ought to give them awareness of their special skills, talents, and high-quality features. It needs to spotlight what is brilliant about them and what they could deliver to the fictitious function they're auditioning for.

Give the scholars some time to write down what they want as their commercial enterprise. A possible approach for this activity is to have small groups create classified ads for every organization member.

Shared Learning.

That is a simple interest in case you've been having your students write in their journal for the complete term.

Inform the scholars to leaf through their mag entries and reflect. Have them choose one aspect they have got determined out about themselves inside the path of this time period.

While every pupil has decided on some factor, they would really like, sit in a circle and have every pupil proportion out on what they located out over the past three months

Write yourself a Letter

That is every other interest this is suitable for older kids as it calls for pretty superior writing skills.

Inform the students that they'll be writing a letter to themselves, and to be completely honest in view that no person else would be able to look at it.

They could write something they'd like on this letter to their future selves. However, they may need to add in topics that describe their present state.

On every other piece of paper or at the end of this letter, tell college students to write down ten dreams they would like to perform thru the next 12 months.

Have your college students seal the letter and their desires in an envelope, deal with the envelope to each person, and keep it confidential. In three hundred and sixty-five days, mail the letters out to the students.

This is a great feat also a way to inspire your college students to recall how they alternate over time and the way they live identical.

Drawing Self portraits

Make sure that each pupil has get entry to a mirror for this interest. If there isn't one accessible on your classroom, bring a few small mirrors in for the scholars to use.

Inform your students to apply the reflection on drawing a photo of themselves. It doesn't should look exactly like them, but it should be a great representation of them.

This easy act can sell the self-mirrored image in college students (beyond the kind that involves a mirror).

To make this act a step further, have them divide the drawing into half—on the left facet, each pupil should draw herself as she sees herself, and at the right facet, he/she should draw herself as she thinks others see her.

Together with this drawing, the students can make an entry in their magazine on the differences between the esteem level of how they see themselves and how they suppose others see them.

THE END

Real life examples, experiences and more germane information you've read. Take to the therapy, advice yourself, be sincere to yourself and keep reminding yourself.

CPSIA information can be obtained
at www.ICGtesting.com
Printed in the USA
LVHW021741090521
686929LV00002B/378

9 781801 387453